I0435710

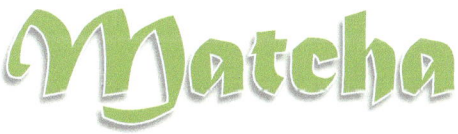

The Key to
Natural Weight
Loss

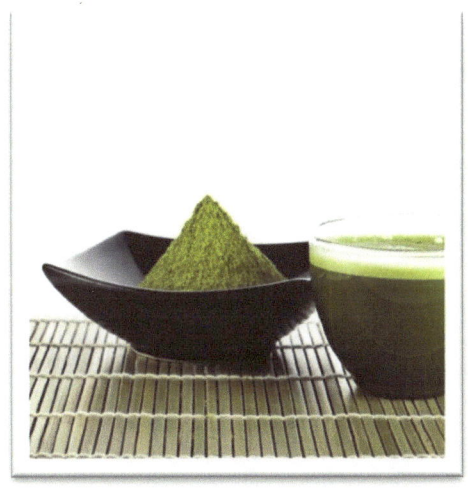

By Rebekah, Lou & Judy Kjos
Holistic Nutritionist & Owners of Got Matcha Premium Tea Co. LLC

ISBN 13: 978-1523432752 EAN-13: 1523432756
Library of Congress Control Number:
pending

Copyright © 2012 by GotMatcha.com
& L.Edward Kjos & Rebekah Winquest
Printed or digitally created
in the United States of America

All rights reserved. No part of this book may be copied or reproduced for
commercial purposes without the written permission of the publisher.

Published by
GotMatcha.com
79 E. Daily Drive #169
Camarillo, CA. 93010

www.GotMatcha.com
Email: info@GotMatcha.com

All information provided by Got Matcha may not be construed as medical
advice or instruction. No action or inaction should be taken based solely
on the contents of this information; instead, readers should consult
appropriate health professionals on any matter relating to their
health and well-being.

Introduction

Matcha, the Ceremonial Green Tea of the ancients, has been a hidden "superfood" to western cultures for a very long time. In the Orient, the knowledge of the incredible benefits of Matcha have been widely known. What has been given little recognition, however, are the wonderful weight loss and weight management benefits found with drinking Matcha on a daily basis. The unique components of Matcha work synergistically together to promote healthy weight loss and weight management.

Matcha brings long-term weight loss compared to most diets and weight loss products. Matcha's ability to cleanse stored fat cells, clear stored waste in the stomach/colon, clean out the arteries and alkalize the body makes Matcha the perfect weight loss superfood because these functions are all essential for long-term weight loss.

The more you implement Matcha into your daily lifestyle, the more your body actually changes to a healthier, stronger fat-burning machine. However, it doesn't just stop there, for as we know, Matcha is a "whole food" that brings a host of benefits beyond "weight loss or weight management".

Matcha helps to handle the stress of daily living, another wonderful benefit, because of the synergistic action of several of it's inherent components, one of which is L-Theanine.

Matcha is truly Mother Nature's answer for the common man. Deal with the stress. Manage the weight. Bring harmony and balance to an overly taxed system. And enjoy life with energy, health and wellness.

Our best to you,

Lou & Judy & Rebekah

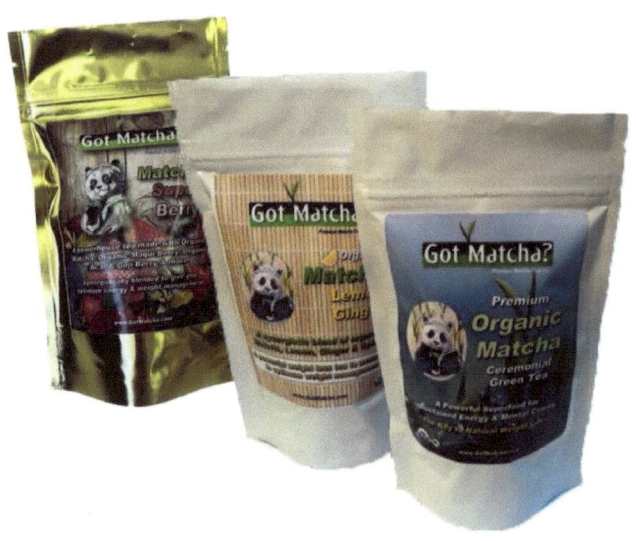

Introducing our "Stars"

Organic Matcha Ceremonial Green Tea
Organic Matcha Lemon-Ginger Tea
Organic Matcha Super Berry Tea

TABLE
OF CONTENTS

Matcha Berry Lemonade
Our latest weight management
powerhouse!

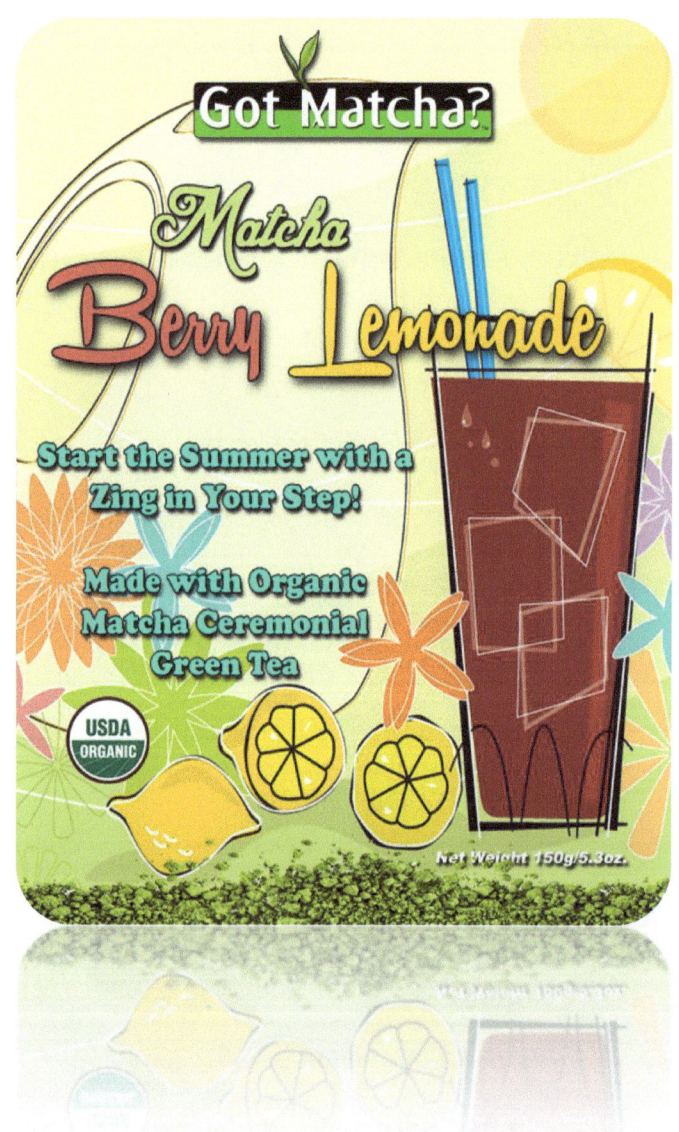

The Matcha Weight Loss Resolution

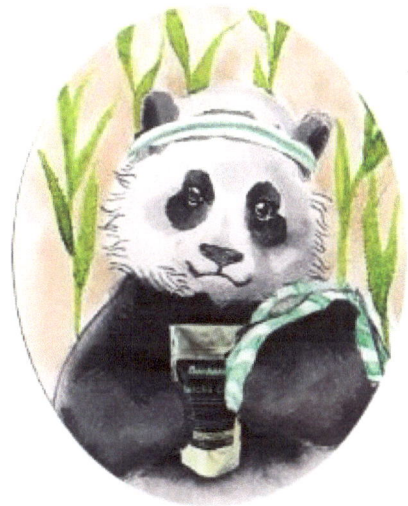

If you could add one new thing to your diet, Matcha green tea should be it if your goal is not only health and energy but healthy weight loss and increased metabolism. Taken 1-3 times/day, Matcha will aid the body in cleansing, elimination, metabolism regulation and pure sustained energy.

- Add Matcha Green tea to a morning shake or drink as tea to aid in cleansing, fat burning, boosting metabolism and energizing the entire body.

- Try drinking 1/2-1 hour after large meals to help digestion.

- Drink Matcha regularly (2-3 times daily) and make sure that one of those cups is within ½ hour before exercising.

- One serving, about ½-1 tsp of Matcha, consumed pre-workout, will help fuel and maintain the body, helping the body to burn more calories and fat.

- Matcha naturally increases your body's energy and heat production during cardio and resistance training which tells the body to burn more calories, specifically fat calories, resulting in weight loss.

- Using Matcha regularly can burn up to four times more calories per workout session.

- Your metabolism can increase as much as 30-40% simply through drinking matcha daily and incorporating it into your workout.

- Matcha is one of nature's best cleansers. Cleansing is key for multiple reasons, and it has a direct affect on weight loss in that you have stored weight in the form of fat cells that have built up in your colon and in abdominal areas. Fat stores in your tissue, skin, around your organs and it all leads to unnecessary toxic weight.

- By drinking Matcha daily, you will be able to cleanse and detoxify your system. You literally clear and filter toxins, stored fat cells and waste products. This process allows your body to work on enhancing its basic functions, especially digestion and daily cleansing. Once your body is clean and working well, you can use or eliminate the food you eat instead of letting it build up as excess weight in your body.

- Matcha keeps the metabolism going throughout the day and keeps you from feeling starved between meals.

- Every morning should start with a Matcha drink for optimal weight loss and weight management. The morning time is your best window to cleanse the stored fats from the previous day along with jumpstarting your metabolism.

Because it is more concentrated and absorbs better into the blood stream compared to traditional steep green tea, Matcha has a greater influence on metabolism, digestion, cleansing, and minimizing the appetite.

Are You New to Matcha?

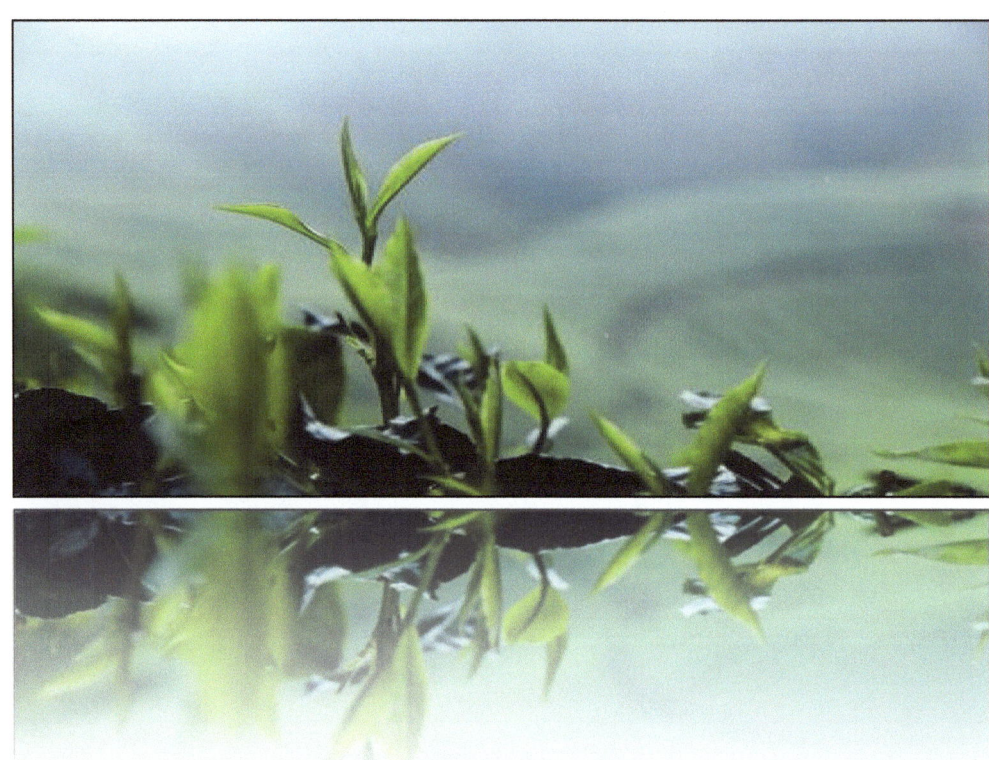

What is Matcha and why should I drink Matcha?

Matcha green tea is known as the "Ceremonial Tea" in Japan and is ritualized in the traditional Japanese tea ceremony that demands a premium and pure tea for overall clarity and to enable focus in meditation. Most immediately, Matcha is an amazing source of energy.

We all operate at different energy levels based on our respective lifestyles and schedules. Matcha has a keen way of not interfering with energy, like coffee or other caffeinated beverages. It flows more naturally—adapting to us rather than requiring us to adapt to it.

Although Matcha is a relative to traditional steeped green tea leaves, this is not your common green tea. You can think of Matcha as a whole food, a premium source packed with so many vitamins, minerals, nutrients, antioxidants and amino acids that it conspires to sustain your body energetically and nutritionally for hours at a time.

Matcha's root function enables sustained energy and endurance, which helps activate the metabolism. More broadly, Matcha is beneficial for those with high blood pressure, and is a cross-functional superfood — battling disorders such as diabetes, obesity, digestive snags—enabling cleansing and regularity, and absolutely can bring your mood out of the depths of minor depression and anxiety—actually providing a natural euphoria without the side-effects of coffee or energy drinks. The most important difference between Matcha and other traditional daily drinks is that it is pure energy, rather than a compromised acidic energy, that is inherent in the coffees and sugar-laced drinks so common in typical commercial cafe. An acidic state wears down the bodily systems over time and sets the body up for failure rather than the success we all strive for (we speak of this further on page 52).

Is the caffeine different from that in coffee and black tea?

The caffeine in Matcha is alkalizing rather than the opposite—acidic. There is caffeine in Matcha, but it releases into the bloodstream slowly. The time of the release varies, but it is not nearly as harsh as the caffeine rush inherent in coffee and energy drinks. This gradual and consistent release provides the body with just the right amount of caffeine over a longer period of time rather than dumping a huge amount of caffeine into the body all at once. Matcha still yields an immediate boost, but not the extreme rush. The lift is far more appropriate to your energy demand, and can be easily regulated based on that demand. Once again, a blast of too much caffeine results in an acidic state that can harm the stomach lining and arteries over time, taxing the organs and disrupting the body's overall functionality. By contrast, Matcha's caffeine has an alkalizing effect, resulting in a much gentler influence on the stomach, which gradually aids with digestion, healing, cleansing. Matcha **gives** to your overall balance rather than taking away.

How does Matcha compare to regular steeped green tea?

Green tea in any form is a source of antioxidants, but Matcha is one of the most powerful sources of antioxidants (catechins & polyphenols), minerals (calcium), trace minerals and Vitamins (A, B-Complex, C, E & K). Why are antioxidants important to our health and longevity? Basically, antioxidants are a preventative; protecting the denaturing of human cells by eliminating free radicals, which are primarily caused by toxins and pollutants. The average American ingests approximately 300 lbs. of chemicals/pollutants/pesticides per year. We are surrounded by chemicals and preservatives in our foods along with toxic gases and carcinogenic chemicals parading through the atmosphere. Matcha is just one source, but one of the most powerful and easily accessed sources, of these critical counters to neutralize daily toxins.

Why does it come in a powder?

Matcha, which means "powdered tea", is made from aged green tea leaves—harvested, steamed and dried. They are later ground into a fine bright green powder, known as Matcha. It is like eating a whole versus a partial food. Unlike other green teas, drinking Matcha is like sucking directly from the leaves and the whole tea plant itself. Therefore, Matcha is much more concentrated in every possible nutrient and more easily absorbed. When common green tea (in a bag) is steeped, only 5-10% of the powerful nutrients are infused into the water. By contrast, Matcha is not steeped, but is a whole plant ground into powder that is blended directly. As such, the powder provides 100% of all the nutrients inherent in the plant.

How should I use Matcha?

It is best to start with ¼-1/2 tsp daily of Matcha and then gradually increase amounts once your body adapts to the tea, up to 1 tsp. 3x/day. We strongly urge those who are new to Matcha not to exceed ½ tsp. of Matcha at a time for the first few weeks because too much at once can be too intense for the body. Like any beverage that naturally stimulates the body, it is wise not to drink on a totally empty stomach until your body has adjusted. We recommend to drink Matcha with milk or add to a smoothie for the first few weeks as you introduce the tea to your system, and not to drink the powder plain with water. Matcha is so rich in powerful nutrients and gentle cleansing properties that there is a chance that someone who is new to this tea may experience minimal nausea.

Here are various ways to prepare your Matcha drink:

- Simply stir in a tea cup of hot milk with a spoon or tea whisk.

- Simply blend the tea with milk and heat over the stove top in a pan.

- Add to a smoothie or to water in a shaker and blend or shake.

- Blend the powder in the blender with about 2/3 cold milk and 1/3 water for a few seconds and then boil it over the stove top in a pan.

- While bringing the milk to a boil in a pan, add the matcha, and then use a whisk and stir constantly while the milk comes to a boil.

What should I expect after drinking it for the first time?

Matcha tea is potent and can have an intense cleansing effect on the body - especially if your body is not used to these types of superfoods. The more toxic build-up you have in your system, the stronger your body may react. Matcha helps to pull the toxins into the blood stream and then filters them out of the body. The side effects can be similar to someone who is implementing a cleanse for the first time. So, like any new practice, proceed with smaller amounts in the beginning to be safe, adapt to your limits, and build up to your energy demand. Enjoy!

Overview
Matcha & Weight Loss

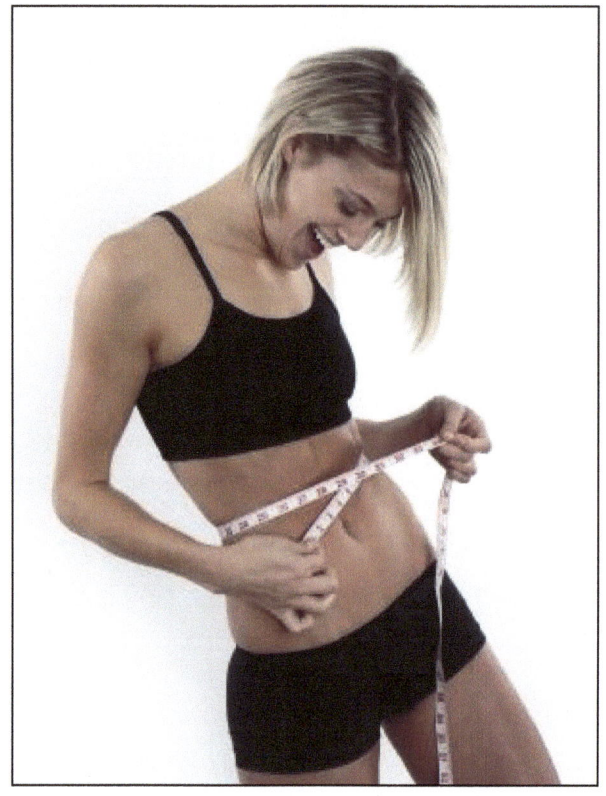

Matcha Green Tea is one of the hidden "superfoods" that has been around for centuries but most people are just now discovering it. It is a super-charged version of regular green tea, and it is an ideal product to facilitate natural and healthy weight loss - *effectively*. Matcha is one of nature's best aids to weight management.

Numerous studies have been done over the past several years concerning the weight loss benefits of drinking green tea; especially Matcha Green Tea.

Matcha green tea assists and literally super-charges your weight loss regime! Why Matcha especially? Because it contains over 10 times the nutritional value of any other green tea and is 10 times or more effective compared to regular green tea for healthy and sustained weight loss!

There are hundreds of weight loss products on the market today claiming to be the missing link to weight loss. You have to be cautious because many products can be harmful to the body's overall health and are not truly natural. Don't waste your money buying green tea tablets for weight loss because Matcha green tea is much more potent and effective for weight loss and increasing your metabolism.

What is great about Matcha is that it is a food that naturally occurs in nature that is harvested, dried, ground into powder and then shipped directly. This is a whole food that not only helps the body reach its ideal weight but is extremely nutritious and healing to the body at the same time.

Daily cleansing with Matcha is key to long term weight loss

The best way to kick off long-term weight loss - and a new lifestyle - is to include a daily regime of Matcha tea in the morning which naturally helps the digestion and cleansing in your body. Cleansing is key for multiple reasons, and it has a direct effect on weight loss in that you have stored weight in the form of fat cells that have built up in your colon and abdominal areas. Fat stores in all your systems including your tissue, skin, around your organs and it all leads to unnecessary toxic weight.

A necessary first step you can take towards natural weight loss is to infuse both a morning matcha drink and an afternoon matcha tea. You will feel some initial energy fluctuation because you are essentially righting the ship and your body will have to adapt to the change. More than not though you will feel a rise in energy because of the fact that digestion takes more energy than any other process, and you are giving the body a rest from digestion allowing the Matcha tea to do all the work. Through cleansing, or detoxification, you clear and filter toxins, stored fat cells and waste products. This process allows your body to work on enhancing its basic functions, especially digestion and daily cleansing. Once your body is clean and working well, you can handle most toxins and use or eliminate the food you eat instead of letting it build up as excess weight in your body.

Get the Most Out of Your Workouts with Matcha Tea

To reach and maintain your overall optimum energy, it is essential to not only eat well, but also to maintain a consistent level of physical activity. This is where Matcha green tea can play an important role. With your workouts, whether your goal is to increase endurance, increase metabolism and/or drop excess visceral fat (the fat stored in the abdominal area), Matcha green tea can assist the body with all three.

The key is to drink Matcha daily. Drinking only 1-2 cups per week of Matcha only before workouts will not allow you to experience the full potential. You will always experience a boost of energy and endurance from one serving of Matcha before a workout but to see results in muscle toning and fat burning, this tea should be drunk on a regular basis.

It is ideal to drink Matcha regularly (2-3 times daily) and when exercising make sure that one of those cups is within ½ hour before exercising. One serving, about ½ to 1 tsp of Matcha, consumed pre-workout will help fuel and maintain the body. Keep in mind that your endurance will increase incrementally over a couple months. You will experience greater energy on a daily basis along with your workouts by the time weeks 8-10 approach with drinking Matcha daily. Various studies have found that physical endurance will improve as much as 20-25% with drinking Matcha on a daily basis and incorporating it into your workouts.

Tip... Did you know that your body is in a state of cleansing from about 4am until 8am? Naturally, your body will be emptier and more cleaned out in the morning than any other time of the day. This is a choice time to engage in physical activity because your body is not preoccupied with digesting a sum of food from the present day. The morning time is ideal for burning those extra stored sugars and fats– your body has less food to burn. I don't advise rolling out of bed, drinking some water and then doing one hour of intense cardio. Your body does need food/energy in some form. Keep it simple. A high-energy and nutrient rich drink, such as a smoothie, with 1 serving of Matcha added.

Why You Should Drink Matcha Every Morning

Your long term weight loss, your energy, and your health, are directly affected by what you put in your body, especially upon waking until noon. What you eat and drink during this time period is crucial and you have the power to mold the rest of your day. Matcha is an alkaline superfood available to us from nature and foods which are alkaline can help balance and heal the body allowing unnecessary stored fats and toxins to be eliminated. Endless research has shown that alkaline foods and drinks in the morning jumpstart the body to burn fuel more efficiently and crave less unhealthy foods throughout the day. Feeding your system alkaline superfoods, like Matcha in the morning, jumpstarts your metabolism for the day, creating the ideal environment for burning and cleansing excess fat cells. As a bonus your body receives good energy and nutrients throughout the day, simply from Matcha.

Think about it, loading up on a high energy drink in the morning like Matcha will not only give you more energy but satisfaction, mental clarity and a happy tummy. The health and sustained weight loss are only a result of what you do on a daily basis – take this daily morning step that can become a ritual.

Increase your metabolism with Matcha

If one of your goals is to increase your metabolism Matcha is one of nature's best and most natural aids. Matcha naturally increases your body's energy and heat production during cardio and resistance training which tells the body to burn more calories, specifically fat calories, resulting in weight loss. Those using Matcha regularly can burn up to four times more calories per workout session.

Studies have found that your metabolism can increase as much as **30-40%** simply through drinking Matcha daily and incorporating it into your workout.

Matcha

Mother Nature's answer to
Natural Weight Management

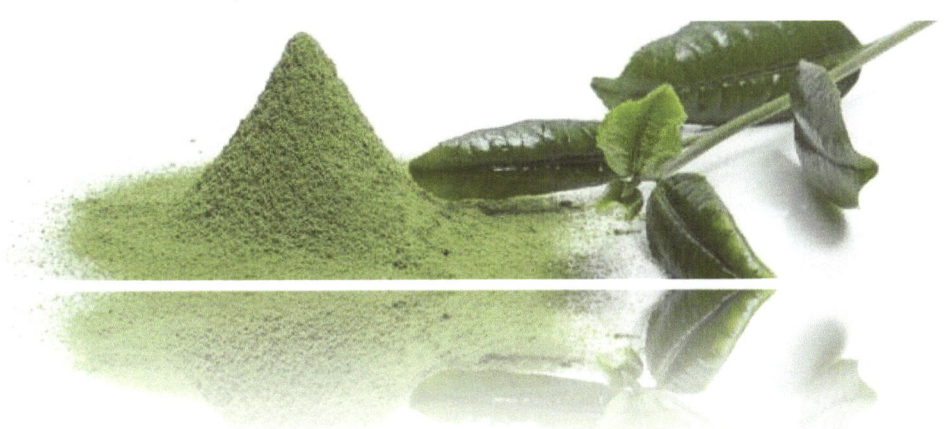

Numerous studies have been done over the past several years concerning the weight loss benefits of drinking green tea; especially Matcha Green Tea. Matcha green tea assists and literally super-charges your weight loss regime! Why Matcha especially? Because it contains over 10 times the nutritional value of any other green tea (one cup of Matcha tea is equivalent to ten cups of steeped green tea)! Matcha drinkers consume the tea plant itself, not just a brew of its leaves. This allows an exponential increase in any health benefits offered including weight loss and boosting the metabolism.

Matcha Green Tea is one of the hidden "superfoods" that people are still discovering. It is a super-charged version of regular green tea, and it is an ideal product to facilitate natural and healthy weight loss - *effectively.*

Weight loss capabilities of Matcha Green Tea:

1. **Metabolism and Matcha:** Green tea speeds up the metabolism, which in turn causes the body to use more calories! Matcha Green Tea also helps to keep the body from storing

excess fat; and it is a natural appetite suppressant. Burn more calories, lose more fat!

2. **Thermogenisis:** Research was conducted in Switzerland about 15 years ago which showed a marked difference in the increase of the metabolism and subsequent burning of calories in a case study done with overweight patients. This process of increasing your metabolism is called "Thermogenesis", which in effect, means that your body's ability to burn off fat is literally supercharged.

3. **Lose Weight Faster:** Replace other drinks with Matcha Green Tea and Lose Weight Faster. An obvious benefit of this plan is to replace the drinks you normally drink with Matcha Green tea; *losing weight will be that much easier!* The average coffee shop drink contains many more calories and grams of fat than you should be drinking just to get the benefit of the caffeine in it.

4. **The Winning Combo:** If you are focused on losing that extra weight, then implementing Matcha Green Tea in conjunction with carefully monitoring what you eat, (and the amounts you eat - like any diet plan), are keystone to a successful weight loss regime.

Losing weight may be only a tea cup away

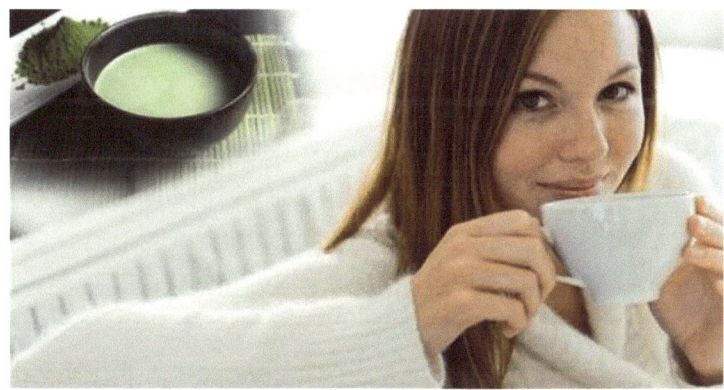

For those looking to shed a few pounds - post-holidays - pre-bikini or simply making healthier lifestyle choices; the solution may be found within a daily cup of Matcha green tea. A part of Zen Buddhist culture for well over 800 years, Matcha is a fine tea powder that is blended and consumed in a drink rather than steeped and discarded like tea leaves.

Clinical research has shown Matcha increases metabolism, offers a huge antioxidant hit and gives a gentle stimulating effect superior to steeped teas.

Weight Loss:

Investigation is on-going concerning the action of Epigallocatechin gallate (EGCG), one of the antioxidants in Matcha, for its potential as an obesity therapeutic with promising results, said Dr. Clifton A. Baile, the CEO of AptoTec, Inc., and a Distinguished Professor of Animal Science and Foods and Nutrition, University of Georgia. Our research has shown that EGCG helps cause weight loss and reduce body fat in mice. There is no magic weight loss solution but, when combined with a healthy lifestyle, drinking Matcha could make losing weight easier.

Published in Obesity Research in June 2005, this study with mouse fat cells showed that EGCG, found in Matcha, helps cause fat cells to store less fat, and eventually, to self-destruct. In a follow-up study not yet published, EGCG fed to mice caused weight loss and reduced the amount of body fat.

The Matcha Alternative:

Negates a Fatty Diet: Most of us have heard of the positive effects red wine can have on a fatty diet and its healthful benefits on heart disease. High amounts of catechins and polyphenols (eg. EGCG) are present in green tea, particularly Matcha tea and EGCG has twice as much resveratrol as red wine, making it a powerful weapon towards lowering cholesterol, inhibiting blood clots and negating the effects of a fatty diet.

Control Your Hunger: EGCG is also used to treat diabetes and is reported to have glucose-lowering effects. In addition, glucose can cause a person to feel hungry, and by controlling insulin levels, you control appetite. Try drinking a mug of Matcha green tea at the first hunger pangs, and you are well on your way to managing your appetite!

In summary, the word thermogenesis literally means heat generation. Matcha Green tea increases thermogenesis in the body, becoming a potent appetite suppressant and increasing fat oxidation. This in turn helps the body to use fat as an energy source. This means the body is preferentially burning fat over protein.

Due to the potency and additional health-promoting properties of Matcha green tea, it is the perfect addition to any weight loss diet or program. Shed pounds in a healthy and effective way!

Matcha
A natural appetite suppressant to curb those cravings!!

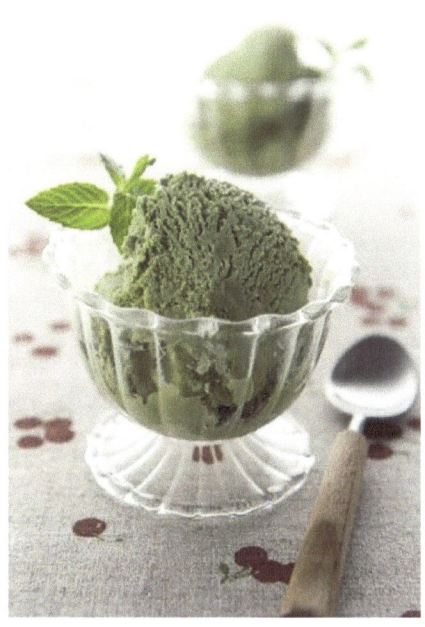

Many weight loss products have to add synthetic and/or extracted ingredients in order to help suppress the appetite. What is great about Matcha is that it naturally helps to control your appetite by telling your brain that you are not hungry in between meals and are full after eating instead of leaving you wanting to overeat. Try drinking Matcha a half hour before larger meals to curb your appetite. Also drink Matcha in between meals to prevent those mid-morning and mid-afternoon munchies.

Most appetite suppressants do only that and provide no other benefits to the body. Matcha on the other hand keeps you from overeating while simultaneously boosting the body with nutrients, antioxidants and sustained energy. Instead of grabbing that sugary, nutrient-empty and calorie-rich latte or soda, replace those drinks with Matcha tea and experience the health benefits while losing weight naturally.

Increase your metabolism with Matcha Ceremonial Green Tea

What is the definition of metabolism?

First understand that everything in life burns energy; whether reading, walking, cleaning or exercising, they all burn energy or calories.

Metabolism measures how many calories your body burns on a daily basis in order to function and maintain itself. There are various factors that contribute to the speed of your metabolism, including age (the older you get the more naturally it slows down), genetics (some people's DNA is more predisposed to burn more on a daily basis) and fitness level. The more muscle you have the more energy your body burns to maintain. Therefore, muscle mass causes the body to burn more calories than fat. You will lose weight via increasing energy output.

How do I increase my metabolism?

If one of your goals is to increase your metabolism, then Matcha is one of nature's best and most natural aids to achieve that goal. Matcha naturally increases your body's energy and heat production, or Thermogenisis, during cardio and resistance training which tells the body to burn more calories, specifically fat calories, resulting in weight loss.

A study featured in the American Journal of Clinical Nutrition found that Matcha green tea produces a significant increase in energy output (a measure of metabolism) in individuals, which is one of the main ways the body loses weight. The study also claimed that Matcha has a significant effect on fat oxidation.

You might think that the weight loss factor is due to the caffeine content in Matcha, however researchers discovered that Matcha green tea's effect on weight loss is only partly attributed to the caffeine. The extra bonus that Matcha adds is its ability to increase thermogenesis in the body. Researchers found that those using Matcha regularly and incorporating it into their workout regime, were able to burn up to four times more calories per workout session, while experiencing an increase in thermogenesis (the body's own rate of burning calories) from a normal 8%-10% of daily energy expenditure to between 35% and 43% of daily energy expenditure. You can anticipate your metabolism to increase by at least 35% simply from drinking Matcha, 1-3 times/day on a daily basis.

Other tips to help increase your metabolism:

- Incorporating exercise is one of the best ways to increase your metabolism. As you build and strengthen your muscles your metabolism increases. You will be burning more at a resting rate, literally, even while sitting down.

- Eat healthy foods and don't starve yourself or follow extreme diets. Not eating enough or often enough actually will slow down your metabolism because your body will go into starvation mode and store the calories. You want to try and eat every 2-4 hours and don't save all of your caloric intake for the end of the day. Don't starve yourself all day and then eat a huge meal at night before bed – that is the perfect formula for fast weight gain and fat storage.

- Keep in mind that once you hit the age of 30 your metabolism naturally slows down a bit. What you were doing in your 20's is most likely not going to be enough. You will need to increase your muscle toning/resistance training, and really be aware of your food choices. You will also need to find other ways to increase your metabolism, such as drinking Matcha.

Matcha and Exercise
Go Hand in Hand

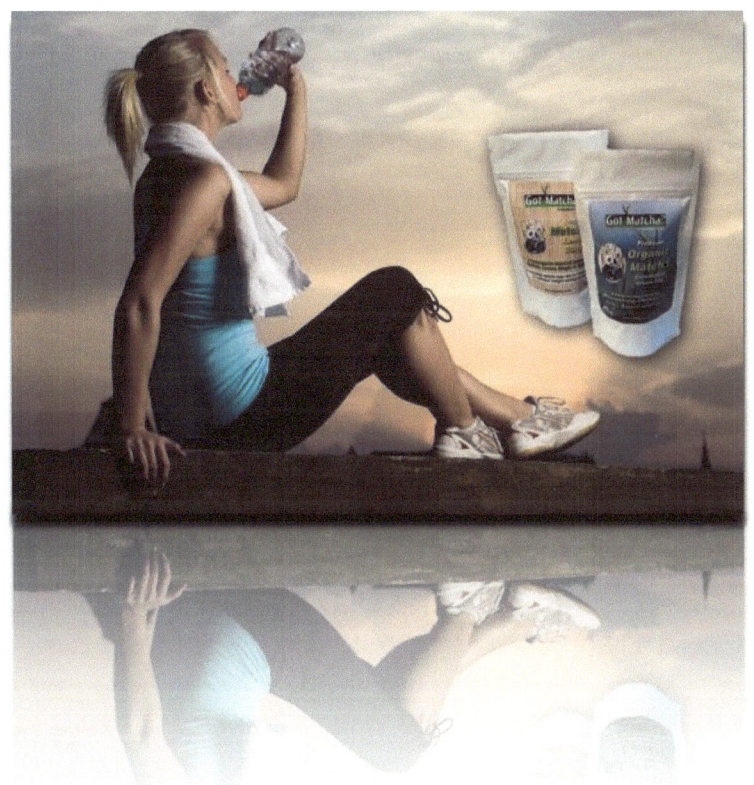

To reach and maintain your overall optimum energy....

It is essential to both eat well and maintain a consistent level of
physical activity. This is where Matcha green tea can play an
important role. With your workouts, whether your goal is to increase
endurance, increase metabolism and/or drop excess visceral fat (the
fat stored in the abdominal area), Matcha green tea can assist the
body with all three.

The key is to drink Matcha daily. I have watched clients drink Matcha
on occasion, only 1-2 cups per week before workouts, and not
understand why they weren't experiencing the full potential. You will

always experience a boost of energy and endurance from one serving of Matcha before a workout but to see results in muscle toning and fat burning, this tea should be drunk on a regular basis.

It is ideal to drink Matcha regularly (2-3 times daily) and make sure that one of those cups is within ½ hour before exercising. One serving, about ½ to 1 tsp of Matcha, consumed pre-workout, will help fuel and maintain the body. Keep in mind that your endurance will increase gradually over a couple months. You will experience more energy on a daily basis along with more stamina and endurance in your workouts by the time weeks 8-10 approach, with drinking Matcha daily. I have read various studies which found that physical endurance will improve as much as 20-25%.

If your goal is weight loss, then next to a healthy diet, Matcha is one of nature's best and most natural aids and is safe for almost every person.

Matcha naturally increases your body's energy and heat production during cardio and resistance training which tells the body to burn more calories, specifically fat calories, resulting in weight loss. Those using Matcha regularly can burn up to four times more calories per workout session. I have found that your metabolism can increase as much as 30-40% simply through drinking matcha daily and incorporating it into your workout.

I personally have been drinking Matcha tea for over 15 years and it not only helps to keep my energy up but it has definitely helped me get rid of those last few post-pregnancy pounds that tend to be a bit stubborn. I encourage all of my clients to drink Matcha regularly and they have not only been able to lose those pounds that love to store abdominally but they experience everything else that Matcha has to offer including energy gain, focus, clarity, immunity and much more.

WHAT TO EAT
FOR YOUR WORKOUT REGIME

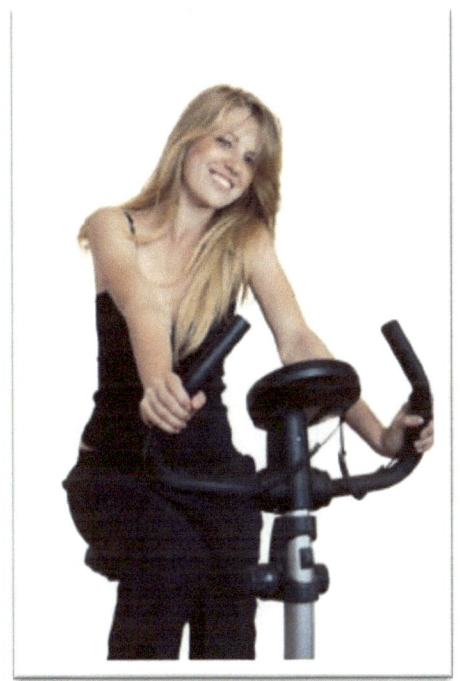

a few suggestions....

I think of exercise less in terms of losing weight, and more in terms of increasing your sustained and balanced energy, which slows down the aging process, and improves your daily life in terms of how you feel. Weight loss is just one of the byproducts of exercise, and should not be the sole focus.

To reach and maintain your overall optimum energy, it is essential to not only eat well, but also to maintain a consistent level of physical activity. Exercising your body brings a balance physically, emotionally and spiritually, and is thus a key to both vitality and rejuvenation. Studies have shown that exercising can reduce your biological age by

10 to 20 years. Foods play an important role with exercise. They can enhance or detract from your workouts. Let's discuss...

- Choosing foods that maximize your endurance & performance levels
- Timing your meals for cardio vs. anaerobic workouts
- Recovery foods

Eating for your workouts

When you start an exercise program, you will want to have an energy strategy to go with it. As I have said, every one of us has a unique body design, and therefore has different energy needs depending on the intensity, goals, and time of day of your workout. No matter what time of day, always follow the 'natural' versus 'processed' guide:

- ❖ Whole grains versus white flour and white rice
- ❖ Raw fats and oils versus fried and saturated oils
- ❖ Natural raw sugars instead of processed white sugar

There are general practices that all of us can follow when preparing the body for a workout. First, you need energy, and energy is created by what you put in your body so regardless of the time of day or intensity of workout, you will want to find the right energy source and should be conscious of how your body will channel that energy.

Here is some helpful advice on the best way to energize for your workout depending on the time of day and the intensity...

<u>**Morning Workout: Before and After**</u>
5 am – Noon

Your body is in a state of cleansing from about 4am until 8am. Naturally, your body will be emptier and more cleaned out in the morning than any other time of the day. This is a choice time to engage in physical activity because your body is not preoccupied with digesting a sum of food from the present day. The morning time is ideal for burning those extra stored sugars and fats—your body has less food to burn. I don't advise rolling out of bed, drinking some water and then doing one hour of intense cardio. Your body does need food-energy in some form. Keep it simple, high-energy and nutrient rich. Here are some examples of foods that I use for my morning energy demand:

- ❖ Green superfood drinks made with coconut water and/or added to a smoothie (don't forget to add your Matcha)
- ❖ Whole sprouted grains (sprouted bread (toast), whole grain/sugar-free cereal, brown rice,
    quinoa) or steel cut oats cooked
- ❖ Dehydrated cookies, cereal or crackers
- ❖ Raw protein like almonds, hemp, walnuts or tempeh
- ❖ Small portion of lean meat or egg whites
- ❖ Vegetables or vegetable juice
- ❖ Starchy fruits like bananas and dates
- ❖ Young Thai Coconuts
- ❖ Raw energy bar

Afternoon Workout
Noon – 5 pm

By the afternoon, you will have probably eaten 2-4 meals (hopefully smaller). If you are planning to work out in the afternoon, adapt your eating schedule so that you have the energy you need for an optimal exercise session. A simple guideline is to eat something the size of your palm, about ½ hour prior to workout, depending on how quickly your body metabolizes food. Focus on the following whole foods and ingredients for sustained good energy:

- ❖ Dehydrated cookies or crackers
- ❖ Complex carbohydrates (whole grains such as brown rice, quinoa)
- ❖ Sandwich with whole grain or spouted bread, veggie, tempeh/tofu or
    lean white meat in a wrap with whole grain tortillas

- ❖ Lean animal or plant-based protein (fish, eggs, tempeh, sunflower seeds, almonds, walnuts, hempseeds, pumpkin seeds)
- ❖ Raw fats (avocado, raw nuts, olive oil, and especially coconut oil)
- ❖ Berries or other raw fruits
- ❖ Salad (vegetables, tempeh, fish, nuts and seeds, olive oil, balsamic vinegar, avocado, sunflower dressing)
- ❖ A second green superfood drink. Or make a smoothie and add a scoop of the green or red superfood powders

Evening Workout

5 pm – 10 pm

It is always challenging to work out in the evening due to a lack of energy, exhaustion after a full work day, or the desire for a big heavy dinner. My recommendations are very similar to the eating habits for an afternoon workout. First, eat a variety of small meals that include whole foods in their natural state every 2-4 hours throughout the day. This will help you keep your energy level up, and help keep you motivated for your workout. Secondly, if you plan to exercise after 6 pm, I advise eating a small good energy meal by 5:30 or 5:45. Here are some examples of quick energy meals to revitalize the body for evening exercise:

- ❖ ½ of a raw superfood/nut bar
- ❖ Fruit sweetened yogurt with raw almonds
- ❖ A small piece of salmon and a handful of baby carrots
- ❖ A slice of sprouted bread with nut butter or coconut oil and honey

After your workout, I wouldn't advise eating a big meal. Keep it simple and light, such as fish and vegetables, humus wrap, tostada, soup, brown rice and vegetables, salad with sprouted bread and avocado.

Timing your Meals

The rule of thumb is to give your body a half-hour to an hour between eating or working out. The time taken is determined by the intensity of your planned workout and what you ate. The digestion of food takes a great deal of energy from your body. Exercise also requires energy. I don't advise eating and exercising simultaneously or within 15 minutes of each other. Let your body digest a bit and then use that energy, which is now filtering throughout your body, for exercise. Raw foods will generally go through your system quicker, about 15-30 minutes. If you have eaten a lot of animal products, give your body at least 30 minutes before engaging in exercise. You can have a green drink 10 minutes before exercising and it should give you great energy.

Low intensity exercises require less pre-digestion time than high intensity. For example, if you are going for a walk, you probably only need about 15 minutes for proper digestion. If you are going to do yoga, aerobics, weight lifting, jogging, or anything that is moderate to high intensity and increases your heart rate above normal, then you want to wait at least 30 minutes.

Tips on Protein Drinks

- Protein Drinks are popular, and are better drunk before or after the workout, not during. Try to allow 15 minutes before or after working out before you have a protein drink. Ideally stick to hemp protein.
- Avoid isolated soy protein because it is processed and toxic.

For those with fast metabolisms

For those of you who digest and burn food very quickly, you may need to eat a larger quantity prior to a workout, and/or bring food for a mid-workout snack. If your blood sugar drops quickly when you exercise, you should pay attention and plan ahead. Eat more complex grains, good fats and lean protein before exercising. Fat provides the body with longer lasting energy, so load up on the almonds, salmon and good raw oils. One tablespoon of raw coconut oil right before a workout has produced amazing results for my family. Coconut oil is raw and un-storable so it circulates energy continuously.

After a workout – Recovery foods & products...
Be kind to your body after exercising. It needs to repair and re-hydrate. Drink lots of alkaline water; eat some lean protein such as:

❖ Fish, tempeh, eggs, raw nuts (almonds, pumpkin seeds, hemp seeds, walnuts)
❖ Healthy raw fats such as avocados, coconut oil, flaxseed oil, raw nuts; whole grain
    breads; grains such as quinoa (extremely high in protein) and brown rice
❖ Vegetables, especially greens
❖ Easily digested protein drinks (hemp protein, rice, or nut based)
❖ Fresh fruit eaten by itself.

It is also beneficial to take a good quality calcium/magnesium after exercising to help relax the muscles and prevent cramping and soreness the next day. The following products can be great for repairing muscles and joints:
❖ MSM
❖ Turmeric
❖ Protein enzymes (Bromelain)
❖ Raw omega fatty acids(flax, fish & hempseed oil)
❖ Ginger
❖ Blue-Green algae ('Blue Mana")

Daily cleansing with Matcha...

A key to long term weight loss

The best way to kick off long-term weight loss, and a new lifestyle, is to include a daily regime of Matcha tea. This will help both digestion and cleansing in your body. Matcha is one of nature's best cleansers. Cleansing is key for multiple reasons, and it has a direct effect on weight loss in that you have stored weight in the form of fat cells that have built up in your colon and abdominal areas. Fat stores in all your systems including your tissue, skin, around your organs and it all leads to unnecessary weight.

Here is how it works...

Your body receives the nourishment your food contains through the absorption of the nutrients as the food travels through the intestines. To properly assimilate these nutrients, the intestinal pathway must be clear. Water cannot flow freely through clogged pipes! It is fairly simple. When the lining of the intestine is blocked by improperly digested food, we receive only minimal benefit and food is more likely to be stored as fat. As surprising as it may seem, overweight people suffer from malnutrition because their intestinal tract is clogged. When our diet includes a variety of plant-based foods, especially superfoods such as Matcha, green grasses and sea vegetables, then we are receiving the proper amount of roughage to help us cleanse stored fats and toxins.

A necessary first step you can take towards natural weight loss is to infuse both a morning Matcha drink and an afternoon Matcha tea.

There are many types of cleansing programs, but what I want to convey is the act of detoxifying and cleansing through foods and/or beverages which can be done daily without having to follow an intense water/juice cleanse. The ideal time to cleanse the body is first thing in the morning with a Matcha drink which helps the body to cleanse stored waste from the previous day. This in turn helps the body prevent fat build up. This practice of a morning detox and energy drink is a total game changer that can help clean your system from the previous day's toxins, and as important, jumpstart you on your day forward. The daily morning detox and energy drink is as important as brushing your teeth, but your systems, just like your teeth, sometimes need a full cleaning.

How should I feel?

You should feel a rise in energy because of the fact that digestion takes more energy than any other process, and you are giving the body a rest from digestion allowing the Matcha tea to do all the work. You should gradually feel less bloated because as the stored fats are cleansed out, your abdominal area will shrink.

This process allows your body to work on enhancing its basic functions, especially digestion and daily cleansing. Once your body is clean and working well, you can handle most toxins and use or eliminate the food you eat instead of letting it build up as excess weight in your body.

Why Matcha?

vs. Extracts and other Weight Loss Products

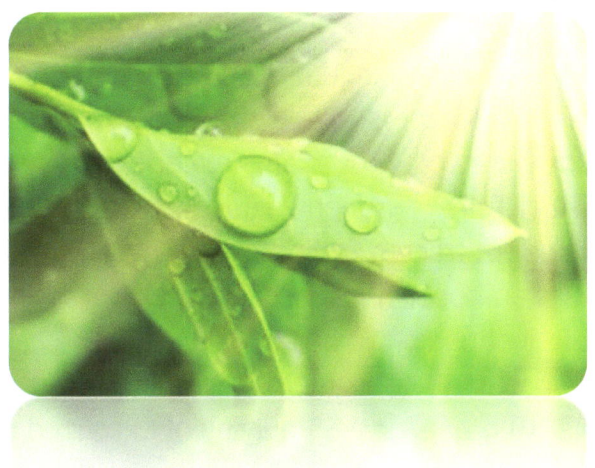

You have to be extremely cautious when it comes to weight loss products. Billions of dollars are spent every year from supplement companies trying to convince consumers to buy their "magic bullet"

weight loss product. The best thing you can do is to be educated about ingredients so that you are not easily swayed towards using products that are in the long run unhealthy and a waste of money.

There is not a magic bullet for weight loss. One pill is not going to remove every pound of excess fat nor will you be able to sustain the weight loss. There are, however, guidelines one can follow. A healthy diet, along with exercise and stress management, help the body to achieve and maintain its optimal weight. Along with a healthy lifestyle, nature has provided many superfoods (a whole food in nature that not only nourishes but can heal and balance the body) that can aid and help facilitate healthy weight loss. Matcha is one such superfood that is rich in vitamins, minerals, antioxidants, specific aminos, and fiber which simultaneously help to rebalance and increase the metabolism, control appetite, cleanse, improve digestion and decrease internal stress; characteristics necessary for healthy weight loss.

GotMatcha's Matcha Lemon-Ginger tea, Matcha Super Berry and our seasonal Matcha Berry Lemonade blends are really the perfect combination for optimal weight loss. The "whole food" ingredients are all natural, nutritious and healing while at the same time work together to enhance your weight loss program.

Most weight loss products contain at least 2 or more ingredients in the form of extracts. An extract is where one part of a whole ingredient is isolated and then extracted. For example, caffeine anhydrous or "caffeine" is pure caffeine commonly added to weight loss pills and drinks that has been extracted from a product that contains caffeine such as tea leaves and poor quality coffee beans. It is also a by-product of decaffeinating coffee beans. Because pure caffeine is toxic, suppliers may not sell it to consumers. According to the FDA, the lethal dose for adults is 10 grams or 0.35 ounces of extracted caffeine, so this is not something to take lightly in a supplement.

Food in nature is does not come in the form of an extract. Foods naturally are made of many components and nutrients and unless you are a scientist you can't extract or isolate one vitamin or mineral from that food. This is why consuming extracted caffeine can be dangerous to one's health because it is too intense and acidic for the body and nature never intended it to be consumed alone versus in a whole food such as tea leaves and Matcha. Yes, Matcha has caffeine but it also contains fiber and other nutrients which work synergistically with the caffeine to help the body absorb it gently without causing harm.

Now let's compare drinking Matcha and/or the Matcha Lemon-Ginger tea to commonly sold weight loss products on the market...

- Many weight loss products add pure caffeine extract to their supplement which can be dangerous for various health conditions, create acidity and will not keep weight off long term.

- The caffeine in Matcha is completely different and unique...it does not harm your internal organs, it does not dehydrate you and because it is found within this whole-food Matcha plant it is released slowly into the bloodstream and regulates the metabolism.

- One weight loss product can contain many ingredients including extracts and ingredients that are not foods but rather act more like a toxin internally, such as Guarana, which contain very high levels of caffeine and cannot be tolerated by those with high blood pressure and heart conditions. It is very acidic and only creates short-term weight loss.

- Matcha is a whole food with nothing else added.

- Most weight loss drinks are sweetened with "sugar-free" sweeteners such as splenda and aspartame which are chemicals *that actually encourage the body to store fat* in the abdominal area.

- Got Matcha teas are sweetened with Stevia and Coconut sugar. Both natural sweeteners do not affect the blood sugar, are not chemicals, and aid in a weight loss regime.

About GotMatcha's
Matcha Lemon-Ginger Tea

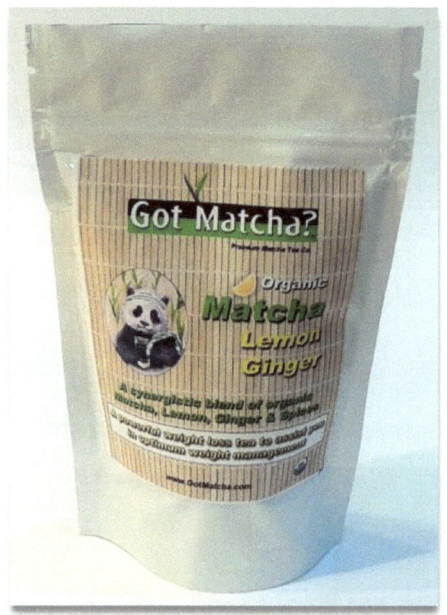

Matcha, alone, is a great natural weight loss tea, however, this new blend of Matcha with lemon peel, ginger and hibiscus takes it one step further. These four-star ingredients work synergistically together to quicken and enhance weight loss properties including cleansing, digestion, boosting metabolism and suppressing appetite.   If you are one that is apprehensive to follow a long extreme juice cleanse, such as the lemon juice, cayenne, and water cleanse; then this tea is ideal. You can still experience the cleansing and weight loss benefits of this tea combined with a healthy diet and moderate exercise.

Let's break down each ingredient in our "Matcha Lemon-Ginger Tea"...

Matcha...

Matcha is one of nature's best aids to weight management. Numerous studies have been done over the past couple of years now concerning the weight loss benefits of drinking green tea; especially Matcha Green Tea.

Hibiscus...

- Mild Diuretic
- Gentle Cleanser

Hibiscus has been know over the years for its ability to act as a mild diuretic which essentially helps to flush out excess water weight. It also works as a gentle laxative aiding the body with cleansing out stored waste and built-up fats. The combination of cleansing out excess fluids and weight stored in the form of fat cells will help to facilitate your weight loss.

Ginger...

- Increases metabolism
- Stimulates digestion
- Reduces bloating and constipation
- Helps lower cholesterol

For centuries Ginger has been recognized for its ability to aid and even tone and strengthen the muscles in the digestive tract. It can motivate over-taxed and inactive livers and it is also able to regulate the spleen and pancreas, which greatly aids digestion. The Chinese believe that the stomach is key to the body's overall state of health. When the digestive tract is working optimally the body is able break down food rather than store it as waste which turns into fat. When the digestive system is functioning at its best, food can move freely through the body, which reduces bloating and constipation.

By keeping the digestive system working more effectively your cholesterol levels can be lowered and maintained because when the veins and arteries have less fatty cells flowing through them cholesterol is less likely to build. Ginger helps to keep your "pipes" clean and flowing freely.

Ginger can increase metabolism because it is able to stimulate various enzymes which can aid metabolism. The better your metabolism, the more calories you will burn.

Lemon Peel...

- Enhances digestion
- Improves bad breathe
- Promotes weight loss

Lemon peel is another gift from nature that has been known for its ability to aid in digestion and even bad breathe because it can destroy bacteria in the intestines and the mouth.

Lemon peel can influence natural weight loss due to its high citric acid content. The citric acid present in lemon peel improves the conversion of stored fat and improves circulation.

How is it sweetened?

Coconut Palm Sugar....the wonder sugar

Coconut Palm sugar is an all-natural, whole food. It contains no chemicals, no additives, no preservatives, no artificial flavors or colorings. It is unrefined and not highly processed as traditional sugars.

Organic Coconut Palm Sugar is derived from the sweet nectar of the sugar blossoms that grow at the top of the tropical coconut palm tree (Cocos Nucifera). Traditional local farmers climb high into the canopy of swaying coconut trees and harvest this sweet nectar by gently slicing open the flower. This nectar is then converted into its traditional crystalline form through boiling the watery sap that drips from the cut flower buds of fresh coconuts.

Coconut Palm Sugar is naturally low on the Glycemic Index (GI), which is important to those who are concerned about weight control and diabetes. Coconut Palm Sugar is rated on the glycemic index at 35, whereas honey is 55 and typical cane sugar is 68.

The low glycemic index of coconut sap sugar is especially helpful as a healthier alternative to those who are pre-diabetic and/or diabetic;

unlike all sugar cane based sweeteners (refined white sugar, brown sugar, muscovado sugar, turbinado sugar, demarara sugar, sucanant sugar, molasses and dehydrated cane juice sweeteners) --- all of which have a high glycemic index rating between 65 to 100 per serving!

Coconut Palm Sugar delivers a slow release of energy, which sustains the human body through the daily activities without experiencing the "highs" and "lows" so often associated with cane sugar. Coconut Palm Sugar also has a nutritional content far richer than any other commercially available sweetener. It is particularly high in Potassium, Magnesium, Zinc and Iron. It is also a natural source of vitamins B1, B2, B3, B6 and C.

Coconut Palm sugar has an exotic flavor profile with wonderful notes of light butterscotch and caramel and add a great flavor profile to our organic Matcha blended teas.

Coconut sugar is a wonderful, nutrient-dense natural sweetener. If we were to define "nutrient dense", it would mean a food that contains a large number of nutrients (eg: vitamins, minerals, amino acids etc) for relatively few calories.

While most sweeteners, especially all artificial and synthetic sweeteners, are devoid of any nutrients, coconut sap sugar is RICH in vitamins, minerals and amino acids. **Coconut sap sugar or palm sugar, is now considered to be one of the best natural sweeteners, being touted as a "wonder sugar" because of its many health benefits**.

How to use this tea for weight loss

GotMatcha's Matcha Lemon-Ginger tea can be enjoyed hot by mixing with milk and water and then heated, or simply by itself. What we have found to be the most effective way to incorporate it into your weight loss regime is to add about 1 Tbsp of the tea blend per 12-16 ounces of cold water and drink throughout the day. Drink a few ounces 15-30 minutes before meals to suppress appetite and help break down the fats in your meal. Drink 15-30 minutes after a meal to increase digestion and aid in cleansing. Drink a few ounces every hour to increase your metabolism and keep your hunger controlled. There is no need to add any milk – tastes great simply mixed with water. Make a double batch in a large water bottle and take it on the go with you throughout the day.

FURTHER KEYS
TO WEIGHT LOSS MANAGEMENT

Weight Loss from the Inside Out

Losing weight is one part of the total strategy for redefining your health. The three topics we will be discussing are:

- Defining your approach to an ideal weight
- The importance of cleansing first
- Essential choices for sustained energy while losing weight

There are base lines that we can refer to when asking the question, "How much should I weigh?" Weight of course is measured in pounds here in America, and the standard ideal weight is calculated from your height, weight, sex, age and frame size. According to this calculation, my ideal weight should be 140 to 160 pounds. I'll be honest with you. That is not my ideal weight.

I want to first discuss the relationship between these two perceptions: "how I look" and "how I feel". The ironic statement by the comedian, Billy Crystal, was such a perfect joke to illustrate a person's obsession on how they look versus how they feel. His character's mantra was, "It's better to look good than to feel good."

In this decade, Billy Crystal's saying of, 'You look maaaarvelous', was invoked by the four New Yorkers in Sex in the City, 'You look faaabulous'. These were two very different contexts, but over time, especially since the onset of emotion driven advertising, the "ideal" has been defined by *how you look* and not *how you feel*.

Now, let me be clear, I want to look good. We all want to look good, but looking good is a very relative perception and it will not define your overall health. My view is that the two perceptions are interdependent, but to keep it simple, we need to approach weight loss with a foundational approach that supports 'how we feel', and how we feel is generally measured by our sustained energy level. For example, are you not able to sleep or is it a struggle to get out of bed in the morning; are you lethargic or depressed throughout the day; is your mental focus blurry or slow; are you motivated to exercise or even walk up the stairs without keeling over? Are you moody or impatient? Examine your energy throughout the day. Where does it drop off? Are you just not performing the physical and mental functions at optimal capacity? Energy should be sustained. It should not be up and down. I feel at my best when my energy is consistent, and when I am living life on purpose with motivation to do more and be more based on my aspirations.

'How you feel' is not only going to be determined by what and when you eat, but how your diet meshes with your total lifestyle, which includes exercise, activities, your environment, workplace stress, sex life, and just the sum of your schedule from day to day. So, to summarize, there is an "ideal weight" for you, but before you define that ideal, you need to discover the right balance to achieve a sustained energy level, and that will be determined by your total lifestyle, and not by a standard calculation or a visual of how you want to look. Billy Crystal was joking. It is much to better to feel good than to look good and my view is that you will look good if you feel good.

The two points I want to make are that first, discuss the importance of cleansing to shed that unnecessary stored weight, and second, to talk about the functional choices you can make in order to sustain your energy level and lose weight simultaneously.

Cleansing and Weight Loss
Cleansing is key for multiple reasons, and it has a direct effect on weight loss in that you have stored weight in the form of fat cells that have built up in your colon and in visceral areas, primarily

around the abdominals and glutes. Fat stores in all your systems including your tissue, skin, around your organs and it all leads to unnecessary toxic weight.

You must eat to lose weight

Eating is important for weight loss – that is eating the right foods! Never cut back your daily intake in an unhealthy way. If you do, you might be slowing down your metabolism, which is what you don't want. If you don't eat for more than 3-4 hours, your metabolism slows down, which creates the environment for storing fat. The body basically thinks that you might not eat again so it creates stores as a contingency. The body is trained to do this so it is critical that you do not allow your body to go into starvation mode. The functional choices you make to replace those dysfunctional choices identified in your choice log should reflect the choices here.

Water

Ideally you should drink, at minimum, half of your body weight in ounces, up to your full body weight in ounces, of alkaline water daily. This helps to rebalance the body, creating the right environment for health, cleansing, and the elimination of acidic fat cells. Your body produces fat cell in order to absorb the acidity in your body but through drinking alkaline water, these cells can be flushed out and the body no longer needs to produce excess fat cells. Plus this water is nutrient rich, keeping the body satisfied

Tip: Try drinking Matcha Lemon-Ginger tea, hot or cold, to to aid digestion and pull bad fats from your body. Try ½ hour before meals.

Start with Superfoods

- Having a daily green drink is essential to nourish, heal, cleanse, and energize the body. This drink should include most of the following: kelp, spirulina, chlorophyll, chlorella, wheat grass, barley grass, oat grass, apple pectin (fiber), flax seed meal, raw hemp seed protein, antioxidant rich berries (red superfoods) and other ground up vegetables.

- Daily green drinks provide the body with a ton of nutrients, which creates less hunger and decreases the "munchies" because the body is so well nourished. Try having your green drink even twice a day to replace a heavier meal.
- I also recommend adding powdered Green Matcha Tea to your green drink for extra energy, cleansing, antioxidants, and a metabolism boost.

50% Raw Foods & Beverages

- Try having green superfood drinks daily.
- Eat lots of leafy greens, sprouts, broccoli, cauliflower, asparagus, carrots, celery, tomatoes, spinach, and bitter greens (kale, collards, chard).
- Try to eat two large salads daily, full of various raw veggies and a light/raw dressing.
- Grapefruit, lemons, apples, papaya and berries great fruits that aid in losing weight.
- Raw Sprouted grains: Try soaking buckwheat and steel cut oats in water over night and eat raw the next morning with nut milk and agave and cinnamon. You can find many brands at the health stores who sell raw, sprouted and dehydrated crackers, cookies, bars, bread, etc. These carbs cannot make you gain weight! They do just the opposite
- Fresh and raw vegetable juice is a great way to fill up on large quantities of nutrients.

Eliminate these choices:

- Alcohol (if you are going to drink, stay with organic wine and use the 1 and 3 rule which means no more than 1 glass a day and no more than 3 glasses in a week.)
- Refined sugar; white flour, including bread or pasta; white rice
- Red meat that is not organic and high fat (still eat minimally or not at all)

- Processed and hydrogenated oil, canola oil, safflower oil, palm oil, vegetable oil, or fried foods including these oils
- Pasteurized dairy products made from cow's milk, especially milk, cream, butter and hard cheese
- Food additives and preservatives such as "Artificial and Natural Flavors
- Refined "table" salt – sea salt only
- Sugar-laden drinks such as soda, pasteurized fruit juice, and most sport drinks which are generally loaded with preservatives and sugar

What to eat minimally or not all

- Try to avoid processed or packaged foods, which include chips, breads, pastas, and basically anything canned, boxed or bagged that has any chemical ingredients added to it!
- Certain carbohydrates, such as refined white flour, or any processed flour, white rice, potatoes, corn and other starches tend to produce more insulin in the body. Even whole wheat flour can raise your insulin levels. The insulin transforms into glucose, or sugar, and when it is not used up, the excess is stored more readily as fat. Avoid those foods during the process of losing weight and definitely minimize thereafter
- If you eat meat, it should be eaten only with vegetables and no more than once daily (fish is the best).

Cooked Grains/Carbs

- The ideal way to eat cooked grains is when they have been sprouted first. The sprouting of the grain predigests the starch, increases the protein and nutrients and makes it easily digested. When cooking grains at home such as brown rice or quinoa, make sure to soak them in water over night before cooking. At health stores there are numerous varieties of already sprouted and baked products such as Ezekiel sprouted bread, pasta, tortillas, etc.

- These carbohydrates, especially brown rice, quinoa, millet, buckwheat, spelt, & amaranth, are a good source of protein and fiber to aid in cleansing the body of stored toxins and accumulated fats.
- Also include cooked fibrous complex carbohydrates such as sprouted yams, and squashes.

Meats

If you choose to eat meat, fish is best, followed by eggs, turkey and chicken. Eat meat once a day at most and have your meat during the day or an early dinner. Try not to combine it with grains and starches – easier to digest if combined only with vegetables.

Legumes (beans)

Legumes are a good source of protein and fiber. They include lentils (which are among the easiest to digest), soybeans, tempeh, chickpeas, white beans, and adzuki beans.

Good Fats

Your body does need "good" fats in the form of Omega Fatty Acids. They can be found in raw nuts, seeds and avocados. Flaxseed oil or meal, hempseed oil and Coconut Oil are good fats that can actually help to pull out the bad fats, make you feel full, and aid in digestion and elimination. Include 1 Tbsp of raw, cold-pressed oils such as Flaxseed, Olive, Coconut and/or Hempseed Oil. About 1-2 grams of Flax seed meal and Hempseed Protein Powder (ground up hemp) is a great addition to cleansing and is a good source of fiber and energy. Olive oil is fine to use in moderation, as long as it is not heated. When trying to lose weight, stick to nuts and seeds that are raw.

Summary of weight loss tips for sustaining your energy while losing weight

- The inclusion of Matcha in your daily regime.
- Green Superfoods (Green Grasses, Algaes, Sea Veggies) -- Satisfies the mind and body's cravings for excess food, due to its nutrient-rich ingredients.
- Drink at least half your body weight in ounces of alkaline water daily.
- Don't skip breakfast – Make sure you drink your greens and eat a couple of small meals by noon. You should eat something within a half hour of waking to get your metabolism going.
- Eat fruit alone. Wait for an hour before eating fruit after a meal; wait 15-30 minutes to eat after fruit.
- Apples are neutral and exceptions to the 'eat fruit alone' rule.
- Avoid eating meat with grains, starches, carbohydrates
- Eat meat only with vegetables
- Green Tea/Matcha Tea -- Keeps metabolism going throughout the day and keeps you from feeling starved between meals.
- Raw/Cold-Pressed EFA's (Essential Fatty Acids), such as Coconut Oil, fish oil, Olive Oil and Flaxseed Oil -- Helps remove bad, stored fats, and fills you up.
- Aloe Vera, Triphala (Ayurvedic Herb) and Flaxseed meal -- cleanses the colon and intestines.
- Raw fiber, including Flaxseed meal, fruit pectin, plant fibers, and Green Grasses – helps the cleansing process and fills you up.
- Probiotics (Acidophilus) – Keeps the colon and intestines free of bacteria and aids in digestion.
- Don't eat too much at one time--eat four to six small meals per day instead of three large meals. Eat a little something (about the size of your palm) every 2-4 hours to keep your metabolism running and to prevent that hungry feeling.

- The majority of your food intake should take place upon waking to about 3 or 4:00 pm. Eat a smaller amount in the evening by 7:00 and only light and raw snacks after 8:00.
- Eat only complex carbohydrates (sprouted whole grains & vegetables) and not simple carbohydrates (sugar, processed/refined flour products including potatoes).
- Exercise – Ideally 1 hour of cardio/yoga/light weights, 4 – 7 times per week, depending on ability and fitness objectives.

The Acid/Alkaline Balance
helping your body maintain a
healthy alkaline balance with
Matcha Green Tea

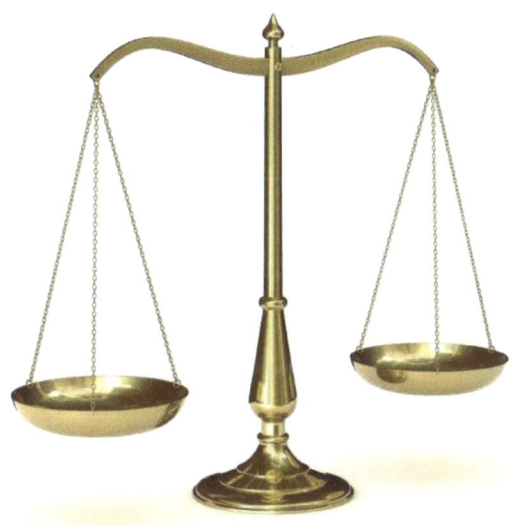

Every aspect of a person's lifestyle synergistically works together to create their "balance", good or bad. There are essential balancing acts within this whole balance, and your PH balance is a primary indicator of that total state of health. Whether your body is in an acid or alkaline state will determine the quality of life you will experience. You may have heard the term "Acidosis". This refers to the condition of your blood and having a PH that is too acidic.

Acidosis is not one specific disease. It is the pre-requisite catalyst and breeding ground for other diseases to develop and be nurtured, such as cancer, osteoporosis, heart disease, high blood pressure, arthritis, obesity, diabetes, allergies, kidney stones, premature aging, and many other degenerative diseases. It is possible to have Alkalosis (too much alkaline), however it is not very common.

<u>Over 90%</u> of the population today is too acidic and has Acidosis.

PH is a measure of how much acid is in the blood. The PH is measured on a scale from 0 to 14 (0 = pure acid and 14 = pure alkaline). Our body strives to be more alkaline, about 7.3 - 7.4. A variant of as little as 2 full points towards acidity, such as 5.3, could be fatal.

The importance of reaching a balanced PH state in the body cannot be emphasized enough. If one truly cares about their quality of life, body, and spirit, then this should be taken very seriously. As mentioned previously, the acidic state is the root of most disease, sickness, and emotional/mental problems.

Scientists have found that cancer thrives in an acidic solution, while it is unable to survive in alkalinity. Just as an embryo grows rapidly and flourishes in the mother's womb surrounded by amniotic fluid, a germ grows quickly and strongly in an acidic environment. By creating an acidic state in our bodies, we are therefore encouraging disease and chaos to be created within. An **inconvenient truth** is that germs are not the source of disease. We create our own harmful & polluted inner environment, which in turn allows the germs to multiply, feed and create their own pollution.

There are a few simple and common factors which disrupt the alkaline balance:

Our thoughts, emotions and stress-levels are very strong factors that are often overlooked when trying to reach alkalinity. They physically create large amounts of acid in our blood when being experienced. *Your thoughts are creative and will have a physical manifestation.* This is a saying that is very true. Stress can cause serious breakdowns and problems within your body no matter how healthy you are eating. That is why stress-management and deep-breathing exercises are so important and can change the state of your body.

All natural foods contain both acid and alkaline forming elements. In some foods, acid-forming elements dominate and vice versa. Such acid-forming foods include animal proteins, cooked oils, alcohol, pasteurized dairy, caffeine, refined/processed grains & carbohydrates, and most cooked nuts & legumes that have not been soaked and/or sprouted first.

Other prevalent factors that induce an acidic state within us are: tap water, most bottled/spring water, distilled water, smog, radiation, pesticides, chemical preservatives, food dye, and additives.

When the blood is overwhelmed with acid ash from foods and stressful emotions, the body relies on a few keys to neutralize acid:

- **When acid is present; the body must then absorb and neutralize it** to become more alkaline. Luckily our bodies are designed with alkaline cell storages, which can soak up the acid to neutralize it. Unfortunately these cells can mutate and become abnormal cells because the acid, during the neutralization process, actually strips the negative charge surrounding the cells. This causes the cells to "glue" together and possibly form malignant/cancerous cells. Simply put, acid could be referred to as glue. Since there are only so many alkaline storages available at a time, the body must use other tactics.

- **Another tactic is for the body to produce fat cells,** which absorb the acid and neutralize it. The unfortunate result creates many unwanted fat cells roaming the body. These cells eventually will lose their respective +/- charges, clump together, and move sluggishly, until they are stored in pockets. This creates excess body fat and lowered energy.

- **The veins and arteries are defenseless culprits of acidic blood**. They are the transport system for the blood to flow throughout the entire body. If the blood running through a vein is highly acidic, a hole could be burned through the vein, allowing the acid to invade the rest of the body. To prevent this, the veins and arteries create and form plaque surrounding the inside walls. This plaque buffers the wall, not allowing the acid to burn a hole. Consequently this self-defense mechanism can be detrimental to one's health. Clogged veins and arteries are precursors to heart attacks, high blood pressure, and many other heart-degenerative diseases.

- **One last common method of protection is the muscles.** Muscle tissues will also absorb and neutralize acid when there is excess for a long period of time. The unfortunate consequence here is that the muscles eventually become "flabby" because the muscle tissues are breaking down. People eating a very acidic diet to lose weight (high-animal protein) are very likely to lose more muscle tone quickly than one who is eating a balanced diet.

There are 4 important steps one can take to reverse the acidic state:

1) **Purchase PH strips**, which can be found at Pharmacies or health food stores. It will have a chart to show you your PH number. Check your PH in the morning before eating. Normal is considered 7.3-7.4, however, above 7 is still considered healthy. The main concern is when your number shows 6.5 and below.

2) **Cleanse** the body of toxins that have developed and taken residence over the years. **Drinking Matcha Green Tea** daily will add to your alkalinity and aid in the cleansing process, including, wheat grass, chlorophyll, green grasses, spirulina, etc. These superfood products are excellent sources of alkaline foods. Matcha specifically will help to cleanse the harmful and disruptive fat cells that have stored up in the body and help to clean out the arteries and colon.

3) Identify choices to create a **target balance of 65%-80% alkaline-forming food**; 20%-35% acidic foods; and about half your body's weight in ounces of well filtered water daily with a PH in the neutral range between 6.5 and 7.5.

The Matcha Challenge
A 7 Day Menu to enhance
your weight loss regime

	1st Thing	Breakfast	Lunch	Snack	Dinner	Snack
Day 1	1 serving (1/2-1 tsp) Matcha tea as a latte heated with milk and water or added to a smoothie	Fruit sweetened yogurt and a handful of raw walnuts or almonds	Salad: lettuce mix, avocado, tomatoes, feta cheese, free-range chicken/tofu /tuna w/ vinaigrette & 3 Tbsp humus w/ 8 rice crackers	Matcha latte or in a shaker cup mix 1 cup coconut water, matcha, almond milk, proten powder	Grilled Salmon, sautéed veggies w/ low sodium Tamari, Coconut/ Grapeseed oil & seasonings	piece of fruit
Day 2	1 serving (1/2-1 tsp) Matcha tea as a latte heated with milk and water or added to a smoothie	Bowl of cooked Steel cut oats with coconut oil, agave or honey and coconut milk	Corn or Ezekiel sprouted tortillas w/ goat cheese; beans or tempeh, veggies, salsa, avocado, lettuce and an apple	Matcha latte or in a shaker cup mix 1 cup coconut water, matcha, almond milk, proten powder	shrimp & veggie stir-fry (try coconut oil, lime juice, cilantro, salt and Tamari) w/ baked squash	bowl of berries
Day 3	1 serving (1/2-1 tsp) Matcha tea as a latte heated with milk and water or added to a smoothie	Spinach/Egg Delight: Saute spinach, garlic, onion, spcices in coconut oil; add whipped eggs and feta	Sprouted bread with humus spread over it topped with tomato, veggies, and raw goat cheese slices from Alta Dena	Matcha latte or in a shaker cup mix 1 cup coconut water, matcha, almond milk, proten powder	Dairy-free vegetarian Soup & quinoa (stir in lemon jiuce, pepper, coconut oil, Celtic Sea Salt and nutritional yeast)	Nana's Gluten free cookie bar (the berry vanilla is delicious)
Day 4	1 serving (1/2-1 tsp) Matcha tea as a latte heated with milk and water or added to a smoothie	Naturally sweetened Yogurt w/ 1/3 cup natural granola	Restaurant Lunch options: Chineese Chicken salad; Simply Grilled Salmon; grilled chicken; or non-dairy soup and salad	Matcha latte or in a shaker cup mix 1 cup coconut water, matcha, almond milk, proten powder	spelt/rice/quinoa pasta w/ tomato sauce & grilled veggies & 4 oz. of fish/ chicken	Raw pudding: Blend banana, peaches/m ango, coconut, vanilla, cinnamon and a handful of raw cashews

Day 5	1 serving (1/2-1 tsp) Matcha tea as a latte heated with milk and water or added to a smoothie	Eggs w/ veggies & goat cheese on a piece of sprouted bread	Turkey Crackers: whole grain long crackers topped w/ goat chevre, dijon mustard & organic turkey slices & handful of baby carrots	Matcha latte or in a shaker cup mix 1 cup coconut water, matcha, almond milk, proten powder	Lg. Asian Salad (chicken, almonds, snow peas, red pepper....Chinese dressing	Young Thai Co onut
Day 6	1 serving (1/2-1 tsp) Matcha tea as a latte heated with milk and water or added to a smoothie	Hot bowl of cooked brown rice w/ honey, cinnamon, raisins & hemp or coconut milk	sandwich with sprouted bread w/ lean chicken/tuna/tempeh, & veggie toppings using Veganaise instead of Mayo	Matcha latte or in a shaker cup mix 1 cup coconut water, matcha, almond milk, proten powder	6 ounces grass fed beef grilled with veggies (Whole Foods will grill for you)	fruit dipped in the raw pudding sauce made from 2 nights before
Day 7	1 serving (1/2-1 tsp) Matcha tea as a latte heated with milk and water or added to a smoothie	Organic frozen gluten-freewaffle toasted almond butter & topped with berries	Sandwich Wrap: In a large sprouted Ezekiel or spelt tortilla spread humus, crumble veggie burger or meat w/ veggies, lettuce, cheese and vinegar	Matcha latte or in a shaker cup mix 1 cup coconut water, matcha, almond milk, proten powder	Black bean tostada (corn tortilla, whole black beans, veggies, salsa, etc.	Non-dairy icecream: try the coconut milk ice cream varieties!

Exercises
You Can Do From Home

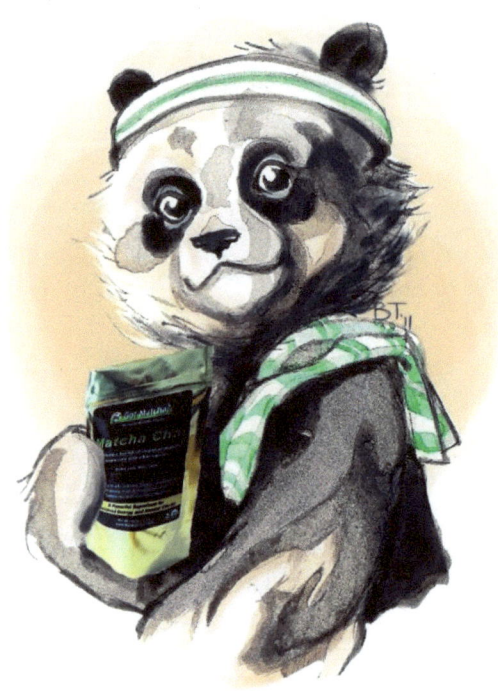

It can be difficult to squeeze workouts in whether you are a stay-at-home parent or a working professional. Regardless of what preoccupies your day you have no excuse not to fit exercises in even if it is only for 5 or 10 minutes at a time...it all adds up and makes a difference. You don't have to go to the gym to workout nor do you have to have warm sunny weather to exercise outdoors. There are many simple exercises that can be done in your home and even in your office.

1. Walking – if it is nice outside go for a walk and if you have kids put them in a stroller walk up hill, you will definitely feel the burn.

2. Jumping Jacks – This is a great way to increase the heart rate and burn extra calories even while watching TV, listening to music or playing with your kids.

3. Pushups are a great way to work the entire body. You don't have to have free weights to tone and strengthen your muscles. Using your body's weight is one of the best ways to work your muscles without over doing it. Pushups work your abs, shoulders, back, arms, glutes, and really every part of the body. You don't have to do pushups traditional style with your toes on the ground. You can do them on your knees, keeping your back straight, against the wall at an angle or even with your hands on an exercise ball while your lower body is straight.

4. Squats – These are one of my favorites and are great for the lower body. They are so versatile and can even be done while brushing your teeth or while you wait for the water to boil. You can do squats with your feet next to each other, with one foot in front and one in the back, walking squats and/or hold light free weights for extra resistance. By holding free weights or even a can of soup in each hand while squatting, the upper body and abs will get a workout too.

5. Abs –
   - Doing simple crunches while lying on your back and bringing your shoulders and arms slightly off the floor and down is a great way to strengthen your stomach muscles.
   - Also try laying on your back with your knees bent and feet on the floor; hold a ball or even a carton of milk between both hands; keep your arms straight and raise slightly off the floor and back down.

- Lay flat on your back, raise your legs straight up in the air and place a light ball, exercise ball or even a water bottle in between your feet and bring them down towards the floor only slightly and back up again.

6. Dancing – Put some music on and dance by yourself or with your kids.

7. Steps – Stepping up and down on a stair, bench or step stool is a great way to tone your leg muscles. Do many repetitions and try adding a squat in between and/or hold free weights.

In conclusion......

Here at GotMatcha, we are very blessed to bring you a wonderful, high quality product in our Organic Matcha and Organic Matcha Lemon-Ginger, Organic Matcha Super Berry, Organic Matcha Berry Lemonade Teas.

They will be your companions for years to come as you continue to maintain a lifestyle that will truly enable your body to heal itself.

Our life is about the choices we make, and adding organic Matcha Ceremonial Green Tea, is just one of those choices that further empowers our ability to live our lives to the fullest.

Best Wishes

Lou & Judy Kjos &
Rebekah Winquest
Got Matcha Premium Tea Co.

www.ingramcontent.com/pod-product-compliance
Lightning Source LLC
Chambersburg PA
CBHW040306010626
45792CB00025B/1141